BLOOD PRESSURE MASTER PLAN:

"The Comprehensive Guide For Combating Hypertension"

OSCAR SYLVAN

stored in a retrieval system, or transmitted in any form or by any means, electronic, mechanical, photocopying, recording, scanning, or otherwise, without the prior written permission of the author.Limit of Liability/Disclaimer of Warranty: This publication is designed to provide accurate and authoritative information in regard to the subject matter covered. It is sold with the understanding that neither the author nor the publisher is engaged in rendering legal, investment, accounting or other professional services. While the publisher and author have used their best efforts in preparing this book, they make no representations or warranties with respect to the accuracy or completeness of the contents of this book and specifically disclaim any implied warranties of merchantability or fitness for a particular purpose. No warranty may be created or extended by sales representatives or written sales materials. The advice and strategies contained herein may not be suitable for your situation. You should consult with a professional when appropriate. Neither the publisher nor the author shall be liable for any loss of profit or any other commercial damages, including but not limited to special, incidental, consequential, personal, or other damages.

Table of Contents

DASH Diet: Dietary Approaches to Stop Hypertension

Key principles of the DASH diet:

Table of Contents

Introduction

About the Author

I am a health enthusiast and writer with a passion for empowering individuals to take charge of their well-being. My own experiences with health challenges have led me to explore holistic approaches to healing and prevention. I believe that true health encompasses not just the absence of disease but also a state of physical, mental, and emotional balance.

Why Holistic Approach Matters

In today's fast-paced world, we often overlook the importance of holistic well-being. We focus on quick fixes and isolated treatments, often neglecting the interconnectedness of our bodies, minds, and spirits. However, a holistic approach to health recognizes that our well-being is a complex interplay of various factors, including our lifestyle, environment, emotions, and spiritual beliefs.

This holistic perspective is particularly important when it comes to managing chronic conditions like hypertension. While conventional medicine plays a crucial role in lowering blood pressure, it often falls short in addressing the underlying causes and the overall impact of hypertension on an individual's life.

Adopting a holistic approach to hypertension management allows us to address the root causes of high blood pressure, such as stress, unhealthy diet, and lack of physical activity. It also encourages us to prioritize emotional well-being, stress management, and

lifestyle modifications that promote overall health and well-being.

Chapter 1

Understanding Hypertension

Definition and Basics

Hypertension, also known as high blood pressure, is a common condition that can lead to serious health problems, including heart disease, stroke, kidney failure, and vision problems. Blood pressure is the force of blood pushing against the walls of your arteries. When your blood pressure is high, it puts extra strain on your heart and blood vessels.

Normal blood pressure is less than 120/80 mmHg. The first number, 120, is your systolic pressure, which is the pressure in your arteries when your heart beats. The second number, 80, is your diastolic pressure, which is

the pressure in your arteries when your heart rests between beats.

High blood pressure is when your blood pressure is consistently 130/85 mmHg or higher. If your blood pressure is high, you may not have any symptoms. However, it is important to get your blood pressure checked regularly, as even mild high blood pressure can increase your risk of serious health problems.

The Importance of Blood Pressure Regulation

Your blood pressure is constantly changing throughout the day in response to various factors, such as physical activity, stress, and sleep. However, your body has a system in place to help regulate blood pressure and keep it within a healthy range. This system includes:

The baroreceptors: These are sensors located in the carotid arteries and aortic arch that detect changes in blood pressure.

The nervous system: The nervous system sends signals to the heart and blood vessels to either increase or decrease blood pressure.

The kidneys: The kidneys help to regulate blood pressure by controlling the amount of fluid in the body.

When blood pressure is not regulated properly, it can lead to hypertension. Many factors can contribute to high blood pressure, including:

Lifestyle factors: These include smoking, obesity, unhealthy diet, lack of physical activity, and excessive alcohol consumption.

Family history: If you have a family history of high blood pressure, you are more likely to develop the condition yourself.

Age: As you get older, your risk of developing high blood pressure increases.

Certain medical conditions: Certain medical conditions, such as diabetes, kidney disease, and sleep apnea, can increase your risk of developing high blood pressure.

Risk Factors and Causes

Many factors can contribute to high blood pressure, but the exact cause is often unknown. Some of the most common risk factors include:

Age: Blood pressure naturally increases with age.

Family history: If you have a parent or sibling with high blood pressure, you are more likely to develop it yourself.

Race: Black adults are more likely to have high blood pressure than white adults.

Obesity: Being overweight or obese increases your risk of high blood pressure.

Diet: A diet high in salt, saturated fat, and cholesterol can increase your risk of high blood pressure.

Lack of physical activity: Exercising regularly can help to lower blood pressure.

Smoking: Smoking can damage your blood vessels and increase your risk of high blood pressure.

Alcohol consumption: Drinking too much alcohol can raise your blood pressure.

Stress: Stress can cause your blood pressure to spike temporarily.

Underlying medical conditions: Certain medical conditions, such as kidney disease, diabetes, and sleep apnea, can increase your risk of high blood pressure.

If you have any of the risk factors for high blood pressure, it is important to talk to your doctor about your risk of developing the condition. Your doctor can help you develop a plan to manage your blood pressure and reduce your risk of serious health problems.

Chapter 2

The Blueprint for Holistic Health

Integrative Medicine and Hypertension

Integrative medicine is an approach to healthcare that focuses on the whole person, mind, body, and spirit. It combines conventional medicine with complementary and alternative medicine (CAM) therapies to provide a comprehensive and personalized approach to healthcare.

Integrative medicine can be an effective way to manage hypertension. Several CAM therapies are beneficial for lowering blood pressure, including:

Acupuncture: Acupuncture is a traditional Chinese medicine technique that involves inserting thin needles into specific points on the body. Studies have shown

that acupuncture can be effective in lowering blood pressure.

Meditation: Meditation is a mind-body practice that involves focusing the mind on the present moment. Studies have shown that meditation can be effective in lowering blood pressure and reducing stress.

Yoga: Yoga is a mind-body practice that combines physical postures, breathing exercises, and meditation. Studies have shown that yoga can be effective in lowering blood pressure and improving overall health.

The Mind-Body Connection

The mind and body are interconnected, and stress can have a significant impact on blood pressure. When we are stressed, our bodies release hormones that can cause our blood pressure to rise. Chronic stress can also contribute to high blood pressure.

There are several things we can do to manage stress and improve our mental health, including:

Exercise: Regular physical activity can help to reduce stress and improve mood.

Relaxation techniques: Relaxation techniques such as yoga, meditation, and deep breathing can help to reduce stress and lower blood pressure.

Social support: Having strong social connections can help to buffer the effects of stress.

Therapy: If you are struggling to manage stress on your own, consider talking to a therapist.

Nutrition and Hypertension

Diet plays an important role in managing hypertension. A healthy diet can help lower blood pressure and reduce the risk of complications from high blood pressure.

Some of the key components of a healthy diet for hypertension include:

Fruits and vegetables: Fruits and vegetables are low in calories and sodium and high in potassium, fiber, and other nutrients that can help to lower blood pressure.

Whole grains: Whole grains are a good source of fiber, which can help to lower blood pressure.

Low-fat protein sources: Low-fat protein sources such as fish, poultry, beans, and tofu are low in saturated fat and cholesterol, which can contribute to high blood pressure.

Limited salt: Too much salt can raise blood pressure. Aim to limit your sodium intake to no more than 2,300 milligrams per day.

Limited alcohol: Alcohol can raise blood pressure. If you drink alcohol, do so in moderation.

In addition to following a healthy diet, several other lifestyle changes can help to lower blood pressure, including:

Quitting smoking: Smoking damages blood vessels and raises blood pressure.

Maintaining a healthy weight: Losing even a small amount of weight can help to lower blood pressure.

Getting regular exercise: Aim for at least 30 minutes of moderate-intensity exercise most days of the week.

Getting enough sleep: Most adults need around 7-8 hours of sleep per night.

By following the tips in this chapter, you can take steps to manage your hypertension and improve your overall health.

Chapter 3

Lifestyle Modifications

Exercise and Physical Activity

Regular physical activity is one of the most important things you can do to lower your blood pressure. Exercise helps to strengthen your heart and lungs, improve blood circulation, and reduce stress. Aim for at least 30 minutes of moderate-intensity exercise most days of the week. This could include activities such as brisk walking, jogging, swimming, or cycling.

Types of exercise

Aerobic exercise: Aerobic exercise is any type of exercise that gets your heart rate up and your blood flowing. Examples include brisk walking, jogging, swimming, cycling, and dancing.

Strength training: Strength training helps to build muscle mass, which can help to lower blood pressure. Examples include lifting weights, using resistance bands, and bodyweight exercises.

Flexibility exercises: Flexibility exercises help to improve your range of motion, which can help to reduce stress and improve circulation. Examples include yoga, Pilates, and tai chi.

How much exercise is enough?

The American Heart Association recommends that adults get at least 150 minutes of moderate-intensity aerobic exercise or 75 minutes of vigorous-intensity aerobic exercise per week. You can also spread this out over the week, doing at least 30 minutes of moderate-intensity exercise most days of the week.

Stress Management Techniques

Stress can contribute to high blood pressure. There are several things you can do to manage stress, including:

Exercise: Exercise is a great way to relieve stress. Aim for at least 30 minutes of moderate-intensity exercise most days of the week.

Relaxation techniques: Relaxation techniques such as yoga, meditation, and deep breathing can help to reduce stress and lower blood pressure.

Mindfulness: Mindfulness involves focusing your attention on the present moment. This can help to reduce stress and improve your overall well-being.

Spending time in nature: Spending time in nature has been shown to reduce stress and improve mood.

Connecting with loved ones: Spending time with loved ones can help to reduce stress and improve your overall well-being.

Sleep and its Impact on Blood Pressure

When you don't get enough sleep, your body produces more of the stress hormone cortisol. Cortisol can raise your blood pressure and make it harder to control. Aim for 7-8 hours of sleep per night.

Tips for getting a good night's sleep

Establish a regular sleep schedule and stick to it as much as possible, even on weekends.

Create a relaxing bedtime routine.

Make sure your bedroom is dark, quiet, and cool.

Avoid caffeine and alcohol before bed.

Get regular exercise, but avoid exercising too close to bedtime.

Additional Lifestyle Modifications

In addition to exercise, stress management, and sleep, several other lifestyle modifications can help to lower blood pressure, including:

Quitting smoking: Smoking damages blood vessels and raises blood pressure.

Maintaining a healthy weight: Losing even a small amount of weight can help to lower blood pressure.

Reducing sodium intake: Too much sodium can raise blood pressure. Aim to limit your sodium intake to no more than 2,300 milligrams per day.

Limiting alcohol intake: Alcohol can raise blood pressure. If you drink alcohol, do so in moderation.

By following the tips in this chapter, you can take steps to lower your blood pressure and improve your overall health.

Please note that these are just general guidelines. It is important to talk to your doctor about what is right for you.

Chapter 4

The Role of Nutrition

DASH Diet: Dietary Approaches to Stop Hypertension

The DASH (Dietary Approaches to Stop Hypertension) diet is a healthy eating plan that can help to lower blood pressure. It is rich in fruits, vegetables, whole grains, and low-fat dairy products. It is also low in saturated and total fat, cholesterol, and sodium.

Key principles of the DASH diet:

Focus on fruits, vegetables, and whole grains: Aim to eat at least five servings of fruits and vegetables and seven servings of whole grains per day.

Choose low-fat dairy products: Limit your intake of full-fat dairy products and choose low-fat or fat-free options instead.

Limit saturated and total fat: Aim to get less than 6% of your calories from saturated fat and less than 25% of your calories from total fat.

Limit cholesterol: Aim to consume less than 200 milligrams of cholesterol per day.

Limit sodium: Aim to consume no more than 2,300 milligrams of sodium per day.

Essential Nutrients for Blood Pressure Regulation

Certain nutrients are essential for regulating blood pressure. These include:

Potassium: Potassium helps to balance the effects of sodium and can help to lower blood pressure. Good sources of potassium include fruits, vegetables, and low-fat dairy products.

Magnesium: Magnesium helps to relax blood vessels and can help to lower blood pressure. Good sources of magnesium include nuts, seeds, and whole grains.

Calcium: Calcium helps to strengthen blood vessels and can help to lower blood pressure. Good sources of calcium include low-fat dairy products, leafy green vegetables, and fortified foods.

Fiber: Fiber helps to lower cholesterol levels and can help to lower blood pressure. Good sources of fiber include fruits, vegetables, and whole grains.

Foods to Avoid

Certain foods can raise blood pressure. These include:

Processed meats: Processed meats are high in sodium and saturated fat, which can raise blood pressure. Examples include bacon, sausage, and ham.

Salty snacks: Salty snacks are high in sodium, which can raise blood pressure. Examples include chips, pretzels, and crackers.

Sugary drinks: Sugary drinks are high in calories and can contribute to weight gain, which can raise blood pressure. Examples include soda, juice, and sports drinks.

Alcohol: Alcohol can raise blood pressure. If you drink alcohol, do so in moderation.

Additional Dietary Tips

In addition to following the DASH diet, several other dietary tips can help to lower blood pressure, including:

Season your food with herbs and spices instead of salt.

Cook your food at home instead of eating out.

Read food labels carefully and choose low-sodium options.

Limit your intake of processed foods.

Drink plenty of water.

By following the tips in this chapter, you can make dietary changes that can help to lower your blood pressure and improve your overall health. Please note that these are just general guidelines. It is important to talk to your doctor or a registered dietitian about what is right for you.

Chapter 5

Herbal Remedies and Supplements

Natural Approaches to Lowering Blood Pressure

Alongside conventional medications and lifestyle modifications, herbal remedies and supplements can offer a complementary approach to managing hypertension. While not intended as a substitute for medical treatment, these natural options may provide additional support for lowering blood pressure.

Herbal Teas and Extracts

Several herbal teas and extracts have shown promise in lowering blood pressure. These include:

Hibiscus tea: Hibiscus tea contains anthocyanins, which have antioxidant and antihypertensive properties. Studies have shown that hibiscus tea can lower both systolic and diastolic blood pressure.

Garlic: Garlic contains allicin, a compound with antihypertensive effects. Studies have shown that garlic supplements can lower blood pressure in people with mild to moderate hypertension.

Olive leaf extract: Olive leaf extract contains oleuropein, a compound with antihypertensive properties. Studies have shown that olive leaf extract can lower blood pressure in people with mild to moderate hypertension.

Hawthorn berry extract: Hawthorn berry extract contains flavonoids, which have antioxidant and antihypertensive properties. Studies have shown that hawthorn berry extract can lower blood pressure in people with mild to moderate hypertension.

Supplement Considerations

Certain supplements may also offer benefits for managing hypertension. These include:

Fish oil: Fish oil contains omega-3 fatty acids, which have anti-inflammatory and antihypertensive effects. Studies have shown that fish oil supplements can lower blood pressure in people with mild to moderate hypertension.

Vitamin D: Vitamin D deficiency has been linked to high blood pressure. Studies have shown that vitamin D supplements can lower blood pressure in people with vitamin D deficiency.

Magnesium: Magnesium deficiency has been linked to high blood pressure. Studies have shown that magnesium supplements can lower blood pressure in people with magnesium deficiency.

Important Considerations

Before incorporating herbal remedies or supplements into your hypertension management plan, it is crucial to consult with your healthcare provider. They can assess your individual needs, potential interactions with existing medications, and appropriate dosage recommendations.

Remember, herbal remedies and supplements should not be considered a replacement for conventional medical treatment. Always prioritize your doctor's guidance and maintain regular checkups to monitor your blood pressure and overall health.

Chapter 6

Mindfulness and Meditation

Mindful Practices for Stress Reduction

Mindfulness and meditation have emerged as powerful tools for managing stress and promoting overall well-being. In the context of hypertension, these practices can play a significant role in lowering blood pressure and reducing the risk of complications.

Mindfulness involves focusing your attention on the present moment, without judgment. This practice can help to break the cycle of stress and anxiety, which can contribute to high blood pressure. Meditation is a form of mindfulness that involves using techniques such as

focusing on the breath or repeating a mantra to achieve a state of mental calmness and clarity.

Benefits of Mindfulness and Meditation

Numerous studies have demonstrated the benefits of mindfulness and meditation for lowering blood pressure. These benefits include:

Reduced stress and anxiety: Mindfulness and meditation can effectively lower levels of stress hormones, such as cortisol, which can contribute to high blood pressure.

Improved emotional regulation: These practices can enhance your ability to manage emotions and cope with stress, further reducing the impact of stress on blood pressure.

Enhanced self-awareness: Mindfulness and meditation promote awareness of your thoughts, feelings, and physical sensations, allowing you to make conscious choices and manage stress effectively.

Guided Meditation Techniques

Guided meditation involves following along with a pre-recorded audio or video instruction, allowing a guide to lead you through the practice. This can be a helpful approach for beginners or those who prefer structured guidance.

Several guided meditation techniques are available specifically for hypertension management. These techniques often focus on relaxation, stress reduction, and promoting feelings of calmness and peace.

Yoga and Tai Chi for Hypertension

Yoga and tai chi are mind-body practices that combine physical postures, breathing exercises, and meditation. These practices are effective for lowering blood pressure and improving overall health.

Yoga involves a series of physical postures (asanas), breathing exercises (pranayama), and meditation techniques. Tai chi is a gentle form of exercise that involves slow, flowing movements.

Benefits of Yoga and Tai Chi

Both yoga and tai chi have been shown to offer several benefits for hypertension management, including:

Improved physical fitness: Regular yoga and tai chi practice can improve overall physical fitness, including flexibility, strength, and balance.

Enhanced stress reduction: These practices can effectively reduce stress and anxiety, which can contribute to high blood pressure.

Improved blood circulation: Yoga and tai chi can enhance blood circulation, promoting overall cardiovascular health.

Mindfulness and meditation: Both practices incorporate elements of mindfulness and meditation, further promoting stress reduction and self-awareness.

Integrating Mindfulness and Meditation into Your Routine

Incorporating mindfulness and meditation into your daily routine can be a simple yet powerful way to manage hypertension. Here are some tips for getting started:

Start small: Begin with short meditation sessions, gradually increasing the duration as you become more comfortable.

Find a quiet and comfortable space: Choose a place where you can relax and focus without distractions.

Explore different techniques: Experiment with various mindfulness and meditation techniques to find what works best for you.

Practice regularly: Aim for regular meditation practice, even if it's just for a few minutes each day.

Seek guidance: If you're new to mindfulness or meditation, consider seeking guidance from a qualified instructor or therapist.

Remember, mindfulness and meditation should be considered complementary practices to conventional medical treatment. Always prioritize your doctor's guidance and maintain regular checkups to monitor your blood pressure and overall health.

Chapter 7

Medication and Medical Interventions

Conventional Medications for Hypertension

Conventional medications are often prescribed to manage hypertension and lower blood pressure. These medications work by targeting various mechanisms in the body that contribute to high blood pressure.

Common Types of Hypertension Medications

Diuretics: Diuretics help increase urine production, which helps to remove excess sodium and fluid from the body, reducing blood pressure.

Angiotensin-converting enzyme (ACE) inhibitors: ACE inhibitors block the production of angiotensin II, a hormone that constricts blood vessels and raises blood pressure.

Angiotensin II receptor blockers (ARBs): ARBs block the action of angiotensin II, preventing it from constricting blood vessels and raising blood pressure.

Beta-blockers: Beta-blockers block the effects of adrenaline, a hormone that increases heart rate and blood pressure.

Calcium channel blockers: Calcium channel blockers block the entry of calcium into smooth muscle cells in the blood vessel walls, causing them to relax and lower blood pressure.

Integrative Approaches to Medication

Integrative approaches to medication involve combining conventional medications with lifestyle modifications and complementary therapies to manage hypertension effectively. This approach aims to minimize the need for medication, reduce side effects, and promote overall well-being.

Benefits of Integrative Approaches

Integrative approaches offer several benefits for managing hypertension, including:

Reduced medication dosage: Lifestyle modifications and complementary therapies can help lower blood pressure, potentially reducing the need for high medication dosages.

Decreased side effects: Lifestyle changes and complementary therapies can help manage side effects from medications, improving overall quality of life.

Enhanced overall health: Integrative approaches promote holistic well-being, addressing not only blood pressure but also overall physical, mental, and emotional health.

Monitoring and Managing Side Effects

While conventional medications can effectively lower blood pressure, they may also cause side effects. It's essential to monitor for potential side effects and communicate any concerns to your doctor.

Common Side Effects of Hypertension Medications

Dizziness or lightheadedness

Fatigue or headache

Dry mouth or cough

Muscle aches or cramps

Sexual dysfunction

Tips for Managing Side Effects

Communicate with your doctor: Openly discuss any side effects you experience with your doctor. They may be able to adjust the dosage or switch to a different medication.

Gradual introduction: Start with a low dosage and gradually increase it as tolerated to minimize side effects.

Lifestyle modifications: Lifestyle changes such as regular exercise, stress management, and a healthy diet can help manage side effects and improve overall health.

Complementary therapies: Explore complementary therapies such as acupuncture, massage therapy, or yoga, which may help alleviate side effects and promote relaxation.

Remember, medication should be considered an integral part of a comprehensive hypertension management plan. Always consult with your doctor to determine the appropriate medication and dosage for your individual needs.

Chapter 8

Monitoring and Managing Blood Pressure

Importance of Regular Check-ups

Regular check-ups with your healthcare provider are crucial for monitoring your blood pressure and managing hypertension effectively. These visits allow your doctor to assess your overall health, evaluate your treatment plan, and make necessary adjustments.

Frequency of Check-ups

The frequency of check-ups may vary depending on your individual needs and the severity of your hypertension. For most people with hypertension, regular check-ups are recommended every 3-6 months.

What to Expect During a Check-up

During a check-up, your doctor will typically perform the following:

Take your blood pressure: Blood pressure is usually measured using a sphygmomanometer, an inflatable cuff placed around your arm.

Review your medication: Your doctor will discuss your medication regimen, dosage, and any potential side effects.

Assess your lifestyle: Your doctor will inquire about your lifestyle habits, including diet, exercise, and stress management.

Evaluate risk factors: Your doctor will assess any underlying medical conditions or risk factors that may contribute to your hypertension.

Using Home Blood Pressure Monitors

Home blood pressure monitoring can be a valuable tool for managing your hypertension. It allows you to track your blood pressure regularly, identify potential trends, and take prompt action if necessary.

Benefits of Home Monitoring

Home blood pressure monitoring offers several benefits, including:

Increased awareness: Regular monitoring can help you become more aware of your blood pressure fluctuations and identify patterns.

Early detection: Home monitoring can help detect early changes in blood pressure, allowing for timely intervention.

Improved communication: Home monitoring data can provide valuable information for discussions with your doctor.

How to Use a Home Blood Pressure Monitor

Choose the right monitor: Select a monitor that is easy to use and provides accurate readings.

Follow the instructions carefully: Read the manufacturer's instructions thoroughly to ensure proper use.

Take measurements consistently: Take your blood pressure at the same time each day and follow a consistent routine.

Record your readings: Keep a log of your blood pressure readings, including date, time, and blood pressure values.

Share your readings with your doctor: Discuss your home monitoring results with your doctor during check-ups.

Tracking Progress

Tracking your blood pressure progress is essential for evaluating the effectiveness of your treatment plan. This can be done through home monitoring logs, charts, or smartphone apps.

Benefits of Tracking Progress

Tracking your blood pressure progress offers several benefits, including:

Monitoring trends: Identifying patterns in your blood pressure readings can help you understand factors that affect your blood pressure.

Assessing treatment effectiveness: Tracking progress allows you to evaluate the effectiveness of your medication, lifestyle modifications, and complementary therapies.

Making informed decisions: Tracking progress can inform discussions with your doctor and guide adjustments to your treatment plan.

Remember, regular monitoring and close communication with your healthcare provider are essential for effective hypertension management.

Chapter 9

Building a Support System

Family and Friends

A strong support system of family and friends can play a vital role in managing hypertension and improving overall health. Their encouragement, understanding, and assistance can help you stay motivated, adhere to your treatment plan, and navigate challenges.

Ways to Build Support from Family and Friends

Communicate openly: Discuss your hypertension with your loved ones, explaining the condition, treatment plan, and how they can support you.

Enlist their help: Ask for specific assistance, such as reminders for medication, encouragement for exercise, or help with preparing healthy meals.

Share your struggles: Be open about the challenges you face, such as side effects of medication or difficulty maintaining lifestyle changes.

Involve them in activities: Invite your loved ones to join you for walks, exercise classes, or healthy cooking sessions.

Express gratitude: Appreciate their support and let them know how much they mean to you.

Joining Support Groups

Joining a support group can provide you with a network of individuals who share similar experiences and challenges. These groups offer a safe and supportive environment to exchange information, share coping strategies, and receive encouragement.

Benefits of Support Groups

Reduced isolation: Support groups provide a sense of belonging and reduce feelings of isolation and loneliness.

Shared experiences: Connecting with others who understand your experiences can provide validation and empathy.

Learning from others: Gain valuable insights and strategies from other members' experiences and successes.

Emotional support: Receive encouragement, motivation, and emotional support from peers.

Improved self-management: Enhance your ability to manage your hypertension and make healthy lifestyle choices.

Communicating with Healthcare Professionals

Open and effective communication with your healthcare providers is crucial for successful hypertension management. They are your partners in navigating your condition and making informed decisions about your treatment plan.

Tips for Effective Communication

Ask questions: Don't hesitate to ask questions about your condition, medication, lifestyle changes, or any concerns you may have.

Express your concerns: Openly discuss any concerns or challenges you face, such as side effects, adherence issues, or lifestyle barriers.

Be proactive: Take an active role in your care by providing accurate information, asking for clarification, and seeking additional resources.

57

Collaborate with your team: View your healthcare providers as partners in your care, working together to achieve optimal health outcomes.

Remember, a strong support system can significantly impact your well-being and empower you to manage your hypertension effectively.

Chapter 10

Personal Success Stories

Real-Life Experiences

Personal success stories of individuals who have successfully managed their hypertension provide valuable inspiration and insights for others facing similar challenges. These stories demonstrate that hypertension is a manageable condition and that lifestyle changes, medication adherence, and support can lead to positive outcomes.

Overcoming Challenges

Individuals with hypertension often face various challenges, including side effects from medication, lifestyle adjustments, and emotional stress. However, these success stories highlight the resilience and determination of individuals who have overcome these hurdles and achieved significant improvements in their health.

Inspiring Transformations

The inspiring transformations of individuals who have successfully managed their hypertension showcase the transformative power of lifestyle changes, medication adherence, and self-care. These stories serve as motivation for others to take charge of their health and strive for improved well-being.

Here are a few examples of inspiring personal success stories:

Sarah: Sarah, a 45-year-old woman, was diagnosed with hypertension at the age of 35. Initially overwhelmed by the diagnosis, she decided to take control of her health and embarked on a journey of lifestyle changes. She adopted a healthy diet, incorporated regular exercise into her routine, and learned stress management techniques. With these changes and consistent medication adherence, Sarah was able to lower her blood pressure to a healthy range and experience significant improvements in her overall health.

David: David, a 60-year-old man, struggled with hypertension for years, finding it challenging to maintain a healthy lifestyle and adhere to his medication regimen. With the support of his family and friends, he joined a hypertension support group, where he found encouragement and shared experiences. Inspired by the group members' success stories, David recommitted to his treatment plan and made gradual lifestyle changes. Over time, he achieved remarkable progress in managing his hypertension and improving his overall well-being.

Maria: Maria, a 55-year-old woman, faced the added challenge of cultural barriers in managing her hypertension. With limited English proficiency and a lack of access to culturally appropriate healthcare resources, she struggled to understand her condition and treatment options. Through the help of a community health worker, Maria received culturally sensitive education about hypertension, learned self-management strategies, and connected with a healthcare provider who spoke her language. With this support, Maria was able to effectively manage her hypertension and make informed decisions about her health.

These personal success stories demonstrate the power of individual determination, the importance of support systems, and the effectiveness of comprehensive treatment approaches in managing hypertension. They serve as beacons of hope for others facing similar challenges, encouraging them to take charge of their health and strive for a healthier, happier life.

Conclusion

Recap of Holistic Approach

Managing hypertension requires a holistic approach that addresses the various factors contributing to high blood pressure. This approach encompasses lifestyle modifications, medication adherence, stress management, and emotional well-being.

Lifestyle Modifications:

Dietary changes: Adopt a healthy diet rich in fruits, vegetables, whole grains, and low-fat dairy products, while limiting processed foods, salt, and unhealthy fats.

Regular exercise: Engage in regular physical activity, aiming for at least 30 minutes of moderate-intensity exercise most days of the week.

Stress management: Practice stress-reduction techniques such as meditation, yoga, deep breathing, or spending time in nature.

Maintaining a healthy weight: Achieve and maintain a healthy weight to reduce the burden on your cardiovascular system.

Medication Adherence:

Follow your doctor's instructions: Take your medication as prescribed and at the recommended times.

Understand the benefits: Recognize the importance of medication in managing your hypertension and improving your overall health.

Communicate with your doctor: Discuss any side effects or concerns you have regarding your medication.

Stress Management and Emotional Well-being:

Prioritize self-care: Dedicate time for relaxation, enjoyable activities, and maintaining a healthy sleep routine.

Seek support: Build a strong support system of family, friends, or support groups for encouragement and understanding.

Address mental health concerns: Seek professional help if you experience persistent stress, anxiety, or depression.

The Journey Ahead

Managing hypertension is an ongoing journey that requires consistent effort and self-care. By adopting a holistic approach that combines lifestyle modifications, medication adherence, stress management, and emotional well-being, you can effectively manage your blood pressure, improve your overall health, and live a fulfilling life.

Remember, you are not alone in this journey. Your healthcare providers are there to support you, provide guidance, and make adjustments to your treatment plan as needed. Embrace the holistic approach, take charge of your health, and embark on a path towards a healthier, happier you.